BREAST CANCER: TREATMENTS

AND

PREVENTIVE METHODS

By

KATHERINE NICHOLS

Copyright © by Katherine Nichols 2023. All rights reserved.

This document should not be copied or otherwise reproduced without the publisher's permission.

As a result, the information inside cannot be transferred, stored electronically, or preserved in a database. The document cannot be copied, scanned, or kept in any way without the publisher's permission.

Table of Contents

Note: For the sake of recurrence of the word "**cancer**", an alternative word "**bosom**" is used in some chapters of this book.

INTRODUCTION

Bosom malignant growth emerges in the covering cells (epithelium) of the pipes (85%) or lobules (15%) in the glandular tissue of the bosom. At first, the harmful development is bound to the pipe or lobule where it for the most part causes no side effects and has insignificant potential for spread.

Over the long run, these in situ (stage 0) malignant growths might advance and attack the encompassing bosom tissue then, at that point, spread to the close by lymph hubs or to different organs in the body. On the off chance that a lady kicks the bucket from bosom malignant growth, it is a result of boundless metastasis.

Bosom malignant growth treatment can be exceptionally compelling, particularly when the sickness is recognized early. Therapy of bosom malignant growth frequently comprises a blend of careful evacuation, radiation treatment and drug (hormonal treatment, chemotherapy as well as designated natural treatment) to treat the infinitesimal disease that has spread from the bosom cancer through the blood. Such therapy, which can forestall disease development and spread, accordingly saves lives.

CHAPTER 1

BREAST CANCER AND THE DEGREE OF THE ISSUE

There were more than 2 million ladies determined to have bosom disease and 685 000 passouts around the world. As of the completion of 2020, there were more than 7 million women alive still up in the air to have chest illness in the past 4 to 5 years, making it the world's most unavoidable harmful development. There are more lost handicap changed life years by ladies to bosom malignant growth around the world than some other sort of disease. Bosom malignant growth happens in each nation of the world in ladies at whatever stage in life after pubescence however with expanding rates in later life.

Bosom malignant growth mortality changed little from the 1930s through to the 1970s. Improvements in perseverance began during the 1980s in countries with early distinguishing proof projects joined with various methods of treatment to kill obtrusive sickness.

Who is in danger?

Bosom malignant growth is certainly not a contagious or irresistible infection. Dissimilar to certain malignant growths that have contamination related causes, for example, human papillomavirus (HPV) disease and cervical malignant growth, there are no realized viral or bacterial diseases connected to the advancement of bosom disease.

Roughly 50% of bosom diseases foster in ladies who have no recognizable bosom malignant development risk factor other than direction and maturity. Certain elements increment the gamble of bosom malignant growth including expanding age, heftiness, hurtful utilization of liquor, family background of bosom disease, history of radiation openness, regenerative history, (for example, age that feminine periods started and age at first pregnancy), tobacco use and postmenopausal chemical treatment.

Conduct decisions and related medications that decrease the gamble of bosom disease include:

-Drawn out breastfeeding;

-Ordinary active work;

-Weight control;

-Evasion of unsafe utilization of liquor;

-Evasion of openness to tobacco smoke;

-Evasion of delayed utilization of chemicals;

- And aversion to extreme radiation openness.

Sadly, regardless of whether the possibly modifiable gamble elements could be all controlled, this would just diminish the gamble of creating bosom malignant growth by at generally 30%.

Female orientation is the most grounded bosom disease risk factor. Roughly 0.5-1% of bosom tumors happen in men. The therapy of bosom disease in men follows similar standards of the board with respect to ladies.

Family background of bosom malignant growth expands the gamble of bosom malignant growth, yet most ladies determined to have bosom malignant growth don't have a known family background of the illness. Absence of a known family ancestry doesn't be guaranteed to imply that a lady is at diminished risk.

Certain acquired "high penetrance" quality transformations extraordinarily increment bosom malignant growth risk, the most prevailing being changes in the qualities BRCA1, BRCA2 and PALB-2. Ladies found to have changes in these significant qualities could think about risk decrease procedures like careful evacuation of the two bosoms. Thought of such a profoundly intrusive methodology just worries an exceptionally set number of ladies, ought to be painstakingly assessed thinking about all other options and ought not be surged.

Signs and effects of Cancer

Bosom disease most usually presents as an easy knot or thickening in the bosom. It is vital that ladies finding an unusual knot in the bosom counsel a wellbeing specialist immediately for more than 1-2 months in any event, when there is no aggravation related to it. Looking for clinical consideration at the earliest hint of a potential side effect takes into account more fruitful treatment.

By and large, side effects of bosom disease include:

A bosom knot or thickening; change in size, shape or presence of a bosom;

dimpling, redness, pitting or other adjustment in the skin.

Change in areola appearance or modification, in the skin encompassing the areola; or potentially unusual areola release.

There are many explanations behind bumps to foster in the bosom, the majority of which are not disease. As numerous as 90% of bosom masses are not malignant. Non-dangerous bosom anomalies incorporate harmless masses like fibroadenomas and blisters as well as contaminations.

Bosom disease can be introduced in a wide assortment of ways, which is the reason a total clinical assessment is significant. Ladies with constant irregularities (by and large enduring over one month) ought to go through tests including imaging of the bosom and at times tissue inspecting (biopsy) to decide whether a mass is dangerous (harmful) or harmless.

High level diseases can disintegrate through the skin to cause open bruises (ulceration) yet are not really excruciating. Ladies with bosom wounds that don't recuperate ought to have a biopsy performed.

Bosom diseases might spread to different regions of the body and trigger different side effects. Frequently, the most widely recognized first perceptible site of spread is to the lymph hubs under the arm despite the fact that it is possible to have malignant growth bearing lymph hubs that can't be felt.

Over the long run, carcinogenic cells might spread to different organs including the lungs, liver, cerebrum and bones. When they arrive at these destinations, new malignant growth related side effects, for example, bone torment or cerebral pains might show up.

The most effective method to treat it

Bosom malignant growth treatment can be profoundly powerful, accomplishing endurance probabilities of 90% or higher, especially when the illness is recognized early. Therapy by and large comprises of a medical procedure and radiation treatment for control of the sickness in the bosom, lymph hubs and encompassing regions (locoregional control) and fundamental treatment (hostile to disease drugs given by mouth or intravenously) to treat or potentially diminish the gamble of the malignant growth spreading. Against disease prescriptions incorporate endocrine (chemical) treatment, chemotherapy and at times designated biologic treatment (antibodies).

Previously, all bosom tumors were dealt with precisely by mastectomy (complete expulsion of the bosom). At the point when malignant growths are huge, mastectomy might in any case be required. Today, most of bosom malignant growths can be treated with a more modest technique called a "lumpectomy" or fractional mastectomy, in which just the cancer is eliminated from the bosom. In these cases, radiation treatment to the bosom is for the most part expected to limit the possibilities of repeat in the bosom.

Lymph hubs are taken out at the hour of disease medical procedure for intrusive tumors. Complete expulsion of the lymph hub bed under the arm in the past was believed to be important to forestall the spread of disease. A more modest lymph hub method called "sentinel hub biopsy" is presently liked as it has less inconveniences. It utilizes color as well as a radioactive tracer to find the initial not many lymph hubs to which malignant growth could spread from the bosom.

Clinical therapies for bosom tumors, which might be given previously or after medical procedure, depends on the natural subtyping of the malignant growths. Diseases that communicate with the estrogen receptor (trauma center) or progesterone receptor (PR) are probably going to answer endocrine treatments like tamoxifen or aromatase inhibitors. These meds are taken orally for 5-10 years, and lessen the chance of repeat of these "chemical positive" diseases by almost half. Endocrine treatments can cause side effects of menopause however are for the most part very much endured.

Malignant growths that don't communicate with a trauma center or PR are "chemical receptor negative" and should be treated with chemotherapy except if the disease is tiny. The chemotherapy regimens accessible today are extremely compelling in decreasing the possibilities of malignant growth spread or repeat and are by and large given as short term treatment. Chemotherapy for bosom malignant growth by and large doesn't need emergency clinic affirmation in that frame of mind of complexities.

Bosom tumors may freely overexpress a particle called the HER-2/neu oncogene. These "HER-2 positive " malignant growths are manageable to treatment with designated organic specialists, for example, trastuzumab. These natural specialists are exceptionally compelling yet in addition pricey, in light of the fact that they are antibodies as opposed to synthetic substances. At the point when designated natural treatments are given, they are joined with chemotherapy to make them successful at killing disease cells.

Radiotherapy likewise assumes a vital part in treating bosom disease. With beginning phase bosom malignant growths, radiation can forestall a lady going through a mastectomy. With later stage malignant growths, radiotherapy can lessen disease repeat risk in any event, when a mastectomy has been performed. For cutting edge phases of bosom malignant growth, in certain conditions, radiation treatment might decrease the probability of passing on from the illness.

The adequacy of bosom malignant growth treatments relies upon the full course of treatment. Fractional treatment is less inclined to prompt a positive result.

Challenges

Endurance of bosom disease for something like 5 years after determination goes from over 90% in big league salary nations, to 66% in India and 40% in South Africa. Early identification and treatment has demonstrated fruitful in big time salary nations and ought to be applied in nations with restricted assets where a portion of the standard devices are accessible. The extraordinarily larger part of medications utilized for bosom malignant growth are as of now on the WHO Fundamental Meds Rundown. In this way, major worldwide enhancements in bosom disease can come about because of carrying out what we definitely know works.

Wide range influence

Age-normalized bosom malignant growth mortality in big league salary nations dropped by 40% between the 1980s and 2020. Nations that have prevailed with regards to lessening bosom malignant growth mortality have had the option to accomplish a yearly bosom disease mortality decrease of 2-4% each year. On the off chance that a yearly mortality decrease of 2.5% each year happens around the world, 2.5 million bosom malignant growth passes would be kept away from somewhere in the range of 2020 and 2040.

The procedures for further developing bosom disease results rely upon key wellbeing framework reinforcing to convey the medicines that are as of now known to work. These are additionally significant for the administration of different tumors and other non-harmful noncommunicable illnesses. For instance, having dependable reference pathways from essential consideration offices to region clinics to devoted disease places.

The foundation of dependable reference pathways from essential consideration offices to area emergency clinics to devoted malignant growth communities is a similar methodology as is expected for the administration of cervical disease, cellular breakdown in the lungs, colorectal malignant growth and prostate malignant growth. Keeping that in mind, bosom malignant growth is an "record" illness by which pathways are made that can be followed for the administration of different sicknesses.

World Wellbeing Association reaction

The target of the WHO Worldwide Bosom Disease Drive (GBCI) is to lessen worldwide bosom malignant growth mortality by 2.5% each year, accordingly deflecting 2.5 million bosom disease passes internationally somewhere in the range of 2020 and 2040. Lessening worldwide bosom disease mortality by 2.5% each year would deflect 25% of bosom malignant growth by 2030 and 40% by 2040 among ladies under 70 years old. The three points of support toward accomplishing these goals are: wellbeing advancement for early discovery; convenient conclusion; and exhaustive bosom disease the executives.

By giving general wellbeing schooling to further develop mindfulness among ladies of the signs and side effects of bosom disease and, along with their families, comprehend the significance of early discovery and therapy, more ladies would counsel clinical professionals when bosom malignant growth is first thought, and before any malignant growth present is progressed. This is conceivable even without a trace of mammographic screening that is unfeasible in numerous nations right now.

State funded instruction should be joined with wellbeing specialist training about the signs and side effects of early bosom disease so ladies are alluded to analytic administrations when fitting.

Quick analysis should be connected to compelling disease therapy that in numerous settings requires some degree of particular malignant growth care. By laying out concentrated administrations in a disease office or emergency clinic, involving bosom malignant growth as a model, therapy for bosom disease might be upgraded while further developing administration of different tumors

CHAPTER 2

VARIOUS SORTS OF BREAST CANCER

Bosom Malignant growth is the most well-known cancer on the planet, a determination that will change the existence of around one of every eight ladies.

Bosom disease basically influences postmenopausal ladies beyond 50 years old, however it doesn't extra men altogether, who address around 1% of all instances of bosom malignant growth.

In spite of long stretches of examination and major logical advancement, tragically, the sickness can in any case be hopeless at determination, particularly when distinguished late.

The consequence of an extreme multiplication of cells brought about by a progression of hereditary changes, this sort of disease can foster in any bosom tissue.

Kinds of Bosom Disease

Contingent upon its capacity to spread inside the organic entity and assault organs and tissue far away from the starting place, bosom disease can be:

Harmless assuming that it stays limited to the region of the bosom where it starts, without spreading through the encompassing bosom tissue.

Obtrusive when the neoplasm can relocate through the lymphatic framework and blood and step by step compromise fundamental capabilities.

The most widely recognized essential locales are:

Lobules: milk-delivering bosom organs.

Lactiferous pipes: the conduits that transport the milk from the lobule to the areola.

The phases of the infection

Contingent upon how cutting-edge the infection is, bosom disease can be analyzed as:

Beginning phase: the growth stays confined in the bosom or axillary lymph hubs.

Privately progressed stage: the sickness has spread to the close by tissue and lymph hubs.

Metastatic stage: the essential cancer has colonized different pieces of the body organic entity, prompting optional growth areas.

While the illness is a lot more uncommon among men than it is among ladies, men can regardless experience the ill effects of bosom disease. As per the Italian Malignant growth Exploration Affiliation, "The instances of bosom disease among men address 0.5-1% of the aggregate".

The low number of findings of this malignant growth among men genuinely compares to a more serious level of forcefulness among male patients

Reasons For Breast Cancer

Specialists realize that bosom disease happens when some bosom cells start to unusually develop. These cells partition more quickly than sound cells do and keep on collecting, framing a bump or mass. Cells might spread (metastasize) through your bosom to your lymph hubs or to different pieces of your body.

Bosom disease most frequently starts with cells in the milk-delivering pipes (obtrusive ductal carcinoma). Bosom disease may likewise start in the glandular tissue called lobules (obtrusive lobular carcinoma) or in different cells or tissue inside the bosom.

Analysts have distinguished hormonal, way of life and ecological variables that might expand your gamble of bosom malignant growth. In any case, it's not satisfactory why certain individuals who have no gambling factors foster disease, yet others with risk factors won't ever do. All things considered, bosom disease is brought about by a complicated collaboration of your hereditary cosmetics and your current circumstance.

Acquired bosom disease

Specialists gauge that around 5 to 10 percent of bosom tumors are connected to quality changes through the ages of a family.

Various acquired transformed qualities that can improve the probability of bosom disease have been distinguished. The most notable are bosom disease quality and bosom malignant growth quality 2, the two of which altogether increase the gamble of both bosom and ovarian disease.

Assuming you have major areas of strength for a background marked by bosom disease or different tumors, your primary care physician might prescribe a blood test to assist with recognizing explicit changes in BRCA or different qualities that are being passed through your loved ones.

Consider asking your PCP for a reference to a hereditary guide, who can survey your family wellbeing history. A hereditary instructor can likewise examine the advantages, dangers and limits of hereditary testing to help you with shared independent direction.

Risk elements of bosom malignant growth

A bosom disease risk factor is anything that makes it more probable you'll get bosom malignant growth. In any case, having one or even a few bosom disease risk factors doesn't guarantee you'll foster bosom malignant growth. Numerous ladies who foster bosom disease have no realized gamble factors other than basically being ladies.

Factors that are related with an expanded gamble of bosom disease include:

Being female: Ladies are significantly more likely than men are to foster bosom disease.

Expanding age: Your gamble of bosom disease increments as you age.

An individual history of bosom conditions: Assuming that you've had a bosom biopsy that tracked down lobular carcinoma in situ (LCIS) or abnormal hyperplasia of the bosom, you have an expanded gamble of bosom disease.

An individual history of bosom disease: In the event that you've had bosom malignant growth in one bosom, you have an expanded gamble of creating malignant growth in the other bosom.

A family background of bosom disease: On the off chance that your mom, sister or little girl was determined to have bosom malignant growth, especially early in life, your gamble of bosom disease is expanded.

In any case, most individuals determined to have bosom malignant growth have no family background of the sickness.

Acquired qualities that increment malignant growth risk: Certain quality transformations that increment the gamble of bosom disease can be passed from guardians to kids.

The most notable quality transformations are alluded to as BRCA1 and BRCA2. These qualities can enormously expand your gamble of bosom malignant growth and different diseases, yet they don't make disease inescapable.

Radiation openness: In the event that you got radiation therapies to your chest as a kid or youthful grown-up, your gamble of bosom disease is expanded.

Heftiness: Being hefty expands your gamble of bosom malignant growth.

Starting your period at a more youthful age: Starting your period before age 12 expands your gamble of bosom disease.

Starting menopause at a more seasoned age: Assuming you started menopause at a more seasoned age, you're bound to foster bosom malignant growth.

Having your most memorable youngster at a more seasoned age: Ladies who bring forth their most memorable kid after age 30 might have an expanded gamble of bosom malignant growth.

Having never been pregnant: Ladies who have never been pregnant have a more serious gamble of bosom malignant growth than do ladies who have had at least one pregnancy.

Postmenopausal chemical treatment: Ladies who take chemical treatment drugs that consolidate estrogen and progesterone to treat the signs and side effects of menopause have an expanded gamble of bosom malignant growth. The gamble of bosom disease diminishes when ladies quit taking these prescriptions.

Drinking liquor: Drinking liquor builds the gamble of bosom malignant growth.

CHAPTER 3

THE BREAST CANCER DIAGNOSIS

Specialists frequently utilize extra tests to find or analyze bosom malignant growth. They might allude ladies to a bosom subject matter expert or a specialist. This doesn't imply that she has a disease or that she wants a medical procedure.

These specialists are specialists in diagnosing bosom issues.

Bosom ultrasound: A machine that utilizations sound waves to make pictures, called ultrasound images, of regions inside the bosom.

Demonstrative mammogram: In the event that you have an issue in your bosom, like protuberances, or on the other hand on the off chance that a region of the bosom looks unusual on a screening mammogram, specialists might have you get a symptomatic mammogram. This is a more definite X-beam of the bosom.

Bosom attractive reverberation imaging (X-ray): A sort of body examine that utilizes a magnet connected to a PC. The X-ray output will make nitty gritty pictures of regions inside the bosom.

Biopsy: This is a test that eliminates tissue or liquid from the bosom to be taken a gander at under a magnifying instrument and do serious testing. There are various types of biopsies (for instance, fine-needle goal, center biopsy, or open biopsy).

In the event that bosom malignant growth is analyzed, different tests are finished to see whether disease cells have spread inside the bosom or to different pieces of the body. This cooperation is called orchestrating Whether the disease is just in the bosom, is tracked down in lymph hubs under your arm, or has spread external the bosom decides your phase of bosom malignant growth. The sort and phase of bosom malignant growth lets specialists know what sort of treatment you want.

Breast Cancer Movement

Obviously bosom disease movement is related with inactivation of various different latent oncogenes. The most broadly assessed growth silencer quality, p53, is transformed in roughly 30-half of irregular bosom diseases. Transformations as a rule happen right off the bat in threatening movement. Loss of heterozygosity (LOH) studies have distinguished various chromosomal locales where other latent oncogenes applicable to bosom malignant growth might be found.

Each LOH is found in a differing extent of bosom malignant growths and may show up either early or late in movement. High-grade ductal carcinoma in situ (DCIS) and obtrusive carcinoma have comparative hereditary sores, demonstrating the way that distortions can happen before obtrusive sickness. Direct proof that similar deviations can be gained later in movement comes from an investigation of numerous metastases from a similar patient; different examinations observed that essential obtrusive diseases are portrayed by stamped intratumor heterogeneity for every sore analyzed.

The model we propose to represent these outcomes guesses that various hereditary sores can achieve every aggregate expected for danger (i.e., dysregulated expansion, intrusion, angiogenesis, and so on) and that, for a given growth, no less than one deviant quality for each phenotypic change is stochastically chosen. Organic heterogeneity of bosom disease results from the stochastic obtaining of different hereditary variations. We further suggest that the lymphocytic response in high-grade DCIS might choose for forceful cancer subpopulations fit for getting away from resistant observation. One more part of growth heterogeneity might be the different systems utilized by different cancers to get away from invulnerable reconnaissance.

Breast Cancer Screening

Frequently you ought to get screening and which tests are generally proper.

The U.S Preventive Administrations Team prescribes that ladies ages 50 to 74 have mammograms like clockwork. They suggest that mammography be viewed as in ladies ages 40 to 49 subsequent to assessing the dangers and advantages of this test with a specialist.

Ladies at ages 40 to 44 are prescribed to have the decision to begin yearly mammography. The suggestion for ladies at ages 45 to 54 is to get mammography consistently and that ladies from 55 and more established can change to having a mammogram like clockwork or proceed with yearly screening in the event that they decide or for however long they are healthy.

Different gatherings likewise give proposals with respect to screening, including the American School of Radiology and the General public of Bosom Imaging. Both suggest yearly mammography beginning at age 40. A few global gatherings don't suggest routine populace based evaluating for any age, however rather suggest an individualized methodology.

The contention about screening mammography is connected with the dangers versus the advantages related to it. The advantage of this screening is finding a malignant growth early that could bring about a superior opportunity of a fix. The gamble is a finding that prompts extra tests when disease is absent and the amount of damage those extra tests possess on the patient. In many regions of the planet, the debate around screening mammography is likewise about possibility and expenses. Bosom malignant growths identified by mammography are many times little. Conversely, quickly developing, forceful tumors are all the more normally tracked in the middle between screening mammograms. They are called stretch tumors. Stretch tumors are more forceful than screen-recognized malignant growths and lead to additional passings contrasted with screen-distinguished diseases. They are likewise more habitually tracked down in more youthful ladies.

In the event that you have a higher gamble of creating bosom disease, screening might be suggested at a prior age and more frequently than the timetables recorded previously. A few more seasoned ladies might quit screening sooner or later, particularly assuming they have huge medical issues that limit the length of their life or capacity to go through the actual requests of bosom malignant growth therapy.

There are additionally unique evaluating suggestions by bunches for bosom disease survivors. Rules distributed in JAMA Oncology suggest that mammography be halted for bosom disease survivors aged 75 and more, assuming they are supposed to live under 5 years. In the meantime, they suggest that mammography be gone on for bosom disease survivors aged 75 and more seasoned who are supposed to live over 10 years.

Therefore it is critical to consult with your PCP about bosom malignant growth screening and settle on a proper evaluating plan for you.

There are likewise various suggestions for clinical bosom assessments. A clinical bosom assessment is the point at which a specialist or other medical care proficient carries out an actual assessment of your bosoms to check for irregularities or bumps. The specialist in this field suggests a clinical bosom assessment alongside mammography. Likewise, it isn't required for ladies with a typical gamble of creating bosom disease to be suggested for a clinical bosom assessment, as it is commonly said there is next to no proof that it assists find with breasting malignant growth early when ladies are additionally getting mammograms. Nonetheless, it is noticed that this doesn't mean these assessments ought to never be finished.

At long last, despite the fact that bosom self-assessment has not been displayed to bring down passings from bosom disease, it is vital to get comfortable with your bosoms so you can know about any progressions and report these to the specialist. Malignant growths that are developing all the more rapidly are in many cases tracked down through bosom in the middle of between normal mammograms.

CHAPTER 4

OPTIONS FOR BREAST CANCER TREATMENT

The phase of your bosom disease is a significant consideration in arriving at conclusions about your treatment choices. By and large, the more bosom malignant growth has spread, the greater treatment you will probably require. Yet, different elements can likewise be significant, for example,

Assuming the malignant growth cells have chemical receptors (that is, assuming the disease is trauma center positive or PR-positive).

Assuming the disease cells have a lot of the HER2 protein (that is, assuming the malignant growth is HER2-positive).

In the event that the malignant growth cells have a specific quality transformation (change).

Your general wellbeing and individual inclinations

On the off chance that you have gone through menopause or not, how quick the malignant growth is developing (estimated by grade or different measures) and assuming it is influencing significant organs like the lungs or liver, talk with your PCP about what these variables can mean for your treatment choices.

Treatment of Ductal Carcinoma in Situ (DCIS)

DCIS is viewed as painless or pre-intrusive bosom disease. DCIS can't spread outside the bosom, however it is frequently treated since, in such a case that let be, a few DCIS cells can keep on going through strange changes that make it become obtrusive bosom malignant growth (which can spread).

Much of the time, a lady with DCIS can pick between bosom rationing a medical procedure

(BCS) and basic mastectomy. Be that as it may, once in a while, assuming DCIS is all through the bosom, a mastectomy may be a superior choice. Clinical examinations are being finished to check whether perception rather than medical procedure may be a possibility for certain ladies.

Bosom preserving a medical procedure.

In bosom monitoring a medical procedure (BMP), the specialist eliminates the cancer and a limited quantity of typical bosom tissue around it. Lymph hub evacuation isn't normally required with BMP. It may very well be performed after the primary medical procedure assuming an area of obtrusive malignant growth is found. The possibilities of an area of DCIS containing intrusive disease goes up with growth size and how quick the disease is developing. In the event that lymph hubs are taken out, this is generally finished as a sentinel lymph hub biopsy (SLNB).

In the event that BMP is finished, it is typically trailed by radiation treatment. This brings down the opportunity of the disease returning a similar bosom (either as additional DCIS or as an intrusive malignant growth). BMP without radiation treatment is definitely not a standard therapy, yet it very well may be a possibility for more established ladies, ladies with other huge medical conditions, or ladies who had little areas of poor quality DCIS that were eliminated with enormous enough malignant growth free careful edges.

Numerous ladies with beginning phase bosom malignant growth, similar to DCIS, can pick between bosom rationing a medical procedure (BMP) and mastectomy. The principal benefit of BMP is that a lady keeps the majority of her bosom. A few ladies could stress that having less broad medical procedures could raise their gamble of the disease returning. However, concentrating on following a large number of people for over 20 years shows that when BCS is finished with radiation in ladies with beginning phase malignant growth , endurance is equivalent to having a mastectomy.

Mastectomy

Straightforward mastectomy (evacuation of the whole bosom) might be required assuming the area of DCIS is extremely huge, in the event that the bosom has a few separate areas of DCIS in various quadrants (multicentric), or on the other hand on the off chance that BMP can't eliminate the DCIS totally (that is, the BMP example re-extraction examples actually have disease cells in or close to the careful edges). On the off chance that a mastectomy is required for any of the reasons expressed above, many specialists will do a SLNB alongside the mastectomy since there is a higher opportunity that obtrusive malignant growth may be found. In the event that an area of obtrusive disease is found in the tissue eliminated during a mastectomy, the specialist will not have the option to return and do SLNB later, and subsequently may need to do a full axillary lymph hub analyzation (ALND) all things considered.

Ladies having a mastectomy for DCIS commonly don't require radiation treatment and may decide to have bosom recreation immediately or later.

Chemical treatment after bosom a medical procedure
In the event that the DCIS is chemical receptor-positive (estrogen or progesterone), therapy with tamoxifen (for any lady) or an aromatase inhibitor, for example, exemestane or anastrozole, (for ladies past menopause) for quite a long time after a medical procedure can bring down the gamble of another DCIS or obtrusive malignant growth creating in one or the other bosom. On the off chance that you

have chemical receptor-positive DCIS, examine the explanations behind and against chemical treatment with your primary care physician.

Therapy of Bosom Disease Stages I-III

The phase of your bosom malignant growth is a significant figure arriving at conclusions about your treatment.

Most ladies with bosom disease in stages I, II, or III are treated with a medical procedure, frequently followed by radiation treatment. Numerous ladies likewise get a fundamental medication treatment of some sort (medication that moves to practically all regions of the body). By and large, the more bosom malignant growth has spread, the greater treatment you will probably require. In any case, your therapy choices are impacted by your own inclinations and different informations about your bosom malignant growth, for example,

On the off chance that the disease cells have chemical receptors. That is, assuming the disease is estrogen receptor (emergency room)- positive or progesterone receptor (PR)- positive.

Assuming the disease cells have a lot of the HER2 protein (that is, in the event that the malignant growth is HER2-positive)

What kind of medication treatment(s) might I get?

Chemotherapy

Chemical treatment (tamoxifen, an aromatase inhibitor, or one followed by the other)

Designated drugs, for example, trastuzumab (Herceptin), pertuzumab (Perjeta), or abemaciclib (Verzenio)

Immunotherapy

The sorts of medications that could work best rely upon the growth's chemical receptor status, HER2 status, and different variables.

Nearby treatment (medical procedure and radiation treatment)

Medical procedure is the primary therapy for stage I bosom disease. These tumors can be treated with either bosom monitoring a medical procedure (BMP; once in a while called lumpectomy or fractional mastectomy) or mastectomy. The close-by lymph hubs likewise should be checked, either with a sentinel lymph hub biopsy (SLNB) or an axillary lymph hub analyzation (ALND).

A few ladies can have bosom recreation simultaneously as the medical procedure to eliminate the disease. Be that as it may, in the event that you will require radiation treatment after medical procedure, it is smarter to hold on to get remaking until after the radiation is finished.

Assuming BMP is finished, radiation treatment is normally allowed after a medical procedure to bring down the opportunity of the malignant growth returning to the bosom and to likewise assist with people living longer.

In a different gathering, ladies who are no less than 65 years of age might think about BMP without radiation treatment in the event that coming up next are all evident:

The growth was 3 cm (somewhat more than 1 inch) or less across and it has been eliminated totally.

None of the lymph hubs eliminated contained disease.

The disease is emergency room positive or PR-positive, and chemical treatment will be given.

Radiation treatment given to ladies with these attributes actually brings down the opportunity of the disease returning, yet it has not been displayed to assist them with living longer.

In the event that you had a mastectomy, you are less inclined to require radiation treatment, however it very well may be given relying upon the subtleties of your particular disease. You ought to talk about in the event that you want radiation therapy with your PCP. You may be shipped off to a specialist radiation (a radiation oncologist) for assessment.

Therapy of Stage IV (Metastatic) Bosom Disease

Stage IV tumors have spread (metastasized) past the bosom and close by lymph hubs to different pieces of the body. At the point when bosom malignant growth spreads, it most regularly goes to the bones, liver, and lungs. It might likewise spread to the cerebrum or different organs.

For ladies with stage IV bosom disease, fundamental medication treatments are the primary medicines. These may include:

-Chemical treatment

-Chemotherapy (chemo)

-Designated drugs

-Immunotherapy

A mix of these Medical procedures and additionally radiation treatment might be valuable in specific circumstances (see underneath).

Treatment can frequently contract growths (or slow their development), further develop side effects, and assist a few ladies with living longer. These malignant growths are viewed as hopeless.

Foundational (drug) therapies for stage IV bosom disease

Therapy frequently goes on until the malignant growth begins developing once more or until secondary effects become unsuitable. On the off chance that this occurs, different medications may be attempted. The sorts of medications utilized for stage IV bosom malignant growth rely upon the chemical receptor status, the HER2 status of the disease, and some of the time quality transformations that may be found.

Chemical receptor-positive diseases

Ladies with chemical (estrogen or progesterone) receptor-positive diseases are some of the time treated first with chemical treatment (tamoxifen or an aromatase inhibitor). This might be joined with a designated medication like a CDK4/6 inhibitor, everolimus, or a PI3K inhibitor.

Ladies who haven't yet gone through menopause are frequently treated with tamoxifen or with meds that hold the ovaries back from making chemicals alongside different medications.

Chemical receptor-negative diseases

Chemo is the fundamental therapy for ladies with chemical (estrogen and progesterone) receptor-negative malignant growths, since chemical treatment isn't useful for these diseases.

HER2-positive tumors.

The main treatment given is typically chemotherapy in mix with trastuzumab (Herceptin, different names) and pertuzumab (Perjeta), both HER2 designated drugs. On the off chance that the disease develops, different choices could include:

An immune response drug form.

A kinase inhibitor with an enemy of HER2 drug or with a chemo drug or both
Other HER2 designated drugs with chemo
Chemical treatment may be added to these medication blends assuming that the malignant growth is likewise chemical receptor positive.

HER2-low diseases.

For bosom tumors that are viewed as HER2-low and have spread to far off locales, the neutralizer drug form fam-trastuzumab deruxtecan (Enhertu) may be a choice.

HER2-negative diseases in ladies with a BRCA quality transformation.

These ladies are regularly treated with a designated drug called a PARP inhibitor, for example, olaparib or talazoparib. Chemotherapy medications and chemical medications are likewise exceptionally supportive in treating these diseases.

HER2-negative malignant growths in ladies with a PIK3CA quality change.

Around 30% to 40% of metastatic trauma center positive bosom tumors have a PIK3CA quality transformation. Alpelisib is a designated drug known as a PIK3 inhibitor that can be utilized alongside the chemical medication fulvestrant to treat postmenopausal ladies with cutting edge chemical receptor-positive bosom disease. For this medication to work, there should be a PIK3CA transformation found on a biopsy done on the growth tissue or of the disease cells in the blood (fluid biopsy).

Triple-negative bosom malignant growth (TNBC).

An immunotherapy drug alongside chemotherapy may be utilized in individuals with cutting edge triple-negative bosom malignant growth whose cancer makes the PD-L1 protein. The PD-L1 protein is tracked down in around 1 of every 5 ladies with triple-negative bosom disease. For ladies with TNBC and a BRCA change, drugs called PARP inhibitors (like olaparib or talazoparib) might be thought of.

For bosom diseases in which the malignant growth cells show elevated degrees of quality changes called microsatellite precariousness (MSI) or changes in any of the confound fix (MMR) qualities (MLH1, MSH2, MSH6, or PMS2), immunotherapy with the medication pembrolizumab may be utilized. Pembrolizumab could likewise be a possibility for TNBC that has other quality or protein changes.

For TNBC that has no particular quality or protein changes, chemo alone or the neutralizer drug form sacituzumab govitecan (Trodelvy) may be a choice.

You can find greater therapy subtleties in Therapy for Triple-negative Bosom Malignant growth.

Neighborhood or local therapies for stage IV bosom malignant growth.

Although foundational drugs are the primary therapy for stage IV bosom malignant growth, neighborhood and territorial therapies like a medical procedure, radiation treatment, or provincial chemotherapy are in some cases utilized too. These can assist with treating bosom disease in a particular piece of the body, however they are probably not going to dispose of the entirety of the malignant growth. These therapies are bound to be utilized to help keep or treat side effects or difficulties from the disease.

Radiation treatment and additionally medical procedure may likewise be utilized in specific circumstances, for example,

-At the point when the bosom cancer is causing an open or excruciating injury in the bosom (or chest).

-To treat a few metastases in a specific region, like the cerebrum.

-To help forestall or treat bone breaks

at the point when disease is pushing on the spinal string.

-To treat a vein blockage in the liver

-To give alleviation of agony or different side effects anywhere in the body.

At times, local chemo (where medications are conveyed straightforwardly into a specific region, for example, into the liquid around the mind and spinal cord, called intrathecal chemo) might be helpful too.

Assuming your PCP suggests such nearby or territorial therapies, you actually must figure out the objective — whether it is to attempt to fix the malignant growth or to forestall or treat side effects.

Most ideal ways to forestall bosom malignant growth

Bosom malignant growth. Simply pursuing those words can make numerous ladies stress. Furthermore, that is normal.

Almost everybody realizes somebody contacted by the illness.

Yet, there is a great deal of uplifting news about bosom disease nowadays. Medicines continue to improve, and we know like never before about ways of forestalling the illness. These eight straightforward advances can assist with bringing down the gamble of bosom disease. Few out of every odd one applies to each lady, yet all in all, they can have a major effect.

1. **Hold Weight In line**

It's not entirely obvious in light of the fact that it gets said so frequently, yet keeping a sound weight is significant for everybody. Being overweight can expand the gamble of various malignant growths, including bosom disease, particularly after menopause.

2. **Be Genuinely Dynamic**

Practice is as near a silver slug for good wellbeing as there is. Ladies who practice for no less than 30 minutes daily have a lower hazard of bosom malignant growth. Ordinary activity is additionally one of the most mind-blowing ways of assisting hold with weighting in line.

3. **Eat Your Natural products and Vegetables - and Cutoff Liquor (Zero is Ideal)**

A sound eating regimen can assist with bringing down the gamble of bosom malignant growth. Attempt to eat a ton of leafy foods and cutoff liquor. Indeed, even low degrees of drinking can expand the gamble of bosom disease. What's more, with different dangers of liquor, not drinking is the general most ideal decision for your wellbeing.

4. **Try not to Smoke**

On top of its numerous other wellbeing gambles, smoking causes something like 15 distinct tumors - including bosom malignant growth. In the event that you smoke, attempt to stop as quickly as time permits. Getting benefits is rarely past the point of no return. You can make it happen. What's more, getting assistance with canning twofold your possibilities stopping for good.

5. **Breastfeed, If Conceivable**

Breastfeeding for a sum of one year or more (joined for all kids) brings down the gamble of bosom disease. It additionally has extraordinary medical advantages for the kid. For breastfeeding data or backing, contact your pediatrician, clinic or nearby wellbeing division.

6. **Keep away from Contraception** Pills, Especially After Age 35 or then again Assuming that You Smoke

Anti-conception medication pills have two dangers and advantages. The more youthful a lady is, the lower the dangers are. While ladies are taking contraception pills, they have a somewhat expanded hazard of bosom malignant growth. This chance disappears rapidly, however, in the wake of halting the pill. The gamble of stroke and coronary episode is likewise expanded while on the pill - especially on the off chance that a lady smokes. However, long haul use can likewise have significant advantages, such as bringing down the gamble of ovarian, colon and uterine malignant growths.

Contraception pills likewise forestall undesirable pregnancy, so there's likewise a great deal in support of themselves. In the event that you're extremely worried about bosom malignant growth, staying away from conception prevention pills is one choice to bring down risk.

7. **Stay away from Chemical** Treatment for Menopause

Chemical treatment in menopause ought not be taken a long haul to forestall persistent sicknesses. Concentrates on showing its blended consequences for wellbeing, raising the gamble of certain illnesses and bringing down the gamble of others. Whether estrogen is taken without anyone else or it's joined with progestin, chemicals increment the gamble of bosom malignant growth. Assuming ladies in all actuality do take chemical treatment during menopause, it ought to be for the most limited time conceivable. The best individual to converse with about the dangers and advantages of chemical treatment for menopause is your PCP.

8. **Tamoxifen and Raloxifene for Ladies at High Gamble**

Albeit not usually considered a "solid

conduct," consuming the medications tamoxifen

what's more, raloxifene can extraordinarily bring down the gamble of

bosom malignant growth in lady at high gamble of the sickness.

Supported by the FDA for bosom disease anticipation,

these strong medications can make side impacts,

so

they aren't ideal for everybody. Assuming you believe you're

at high gamble, converse with your PCP to check whether these medications might be ideal for you.

Conclusion

Figure out Your Family Ancestry

Ladies with a solid family background of malignant growth can find exceptional ways to safeguard themselves. That is the reason it's key for ladies to know their family ancestry. You're at higher gamble on the off chance that you have a mother or sister who had bosom or ovarian disease. This hazard is significantly higher in the event that your relative was analyzed at an early age. Having different relatives (counting guys) who have bosom, ovarian or prostate disease likewise raises your gamble. A specialist or hereditary instructor can assist with making sense of your family background of the sickness.

Remember Mammograms

Bosom malignant growth screening with mammography saves lives. It doesn't assist with forestalling malignant growth, yet it can assist with tracking down disease early when it's more treatable.

Most ladies ought to get yearly mammograms beginning at age 40.

Ladies at higher gamble for bosom disease might have to begin getting screened before. It's ideal to converse with a specialist by age 30 about your gamble and whether you'd profit from prior screening.

Since normal bosom self-tests haven't shown to be gainful, they aren't suggested for screening. All things considered, it is vital to know your bosoms. Tell your PCP immediately in the event that you notice any progressions in how your bosoms look or feel.

www.ingramcontent.com/pod-product-compliance
Lightning Source LLC
Chambersburg PA
CBHW050843260726
48660CB00006B/2410